Atkins Diet

Rapid Weight Loss and Unstoppable Energy

Luke Brooks

Table of Contents

Introduction

I would like to thank you for purchasing this book ''21 Day Atkins Diet Challenge – For Rapid Weight Loss and Unstoppable energy'

This diet hasn't been in existence for long, but has proven to be quite successful and popular. Dr. Robert Atkins, a cardiologist, was the creator of the Atkins Diet. The focus of this diet is to identify the different food groups that would be a perfect match for your metabolism. It might sound impossible, but this is the main objective of the Atkins Diet. When Dr. Robert Atkins had begun his research on diets, he had put his patients on a diet that was low in sugar and carbohydrates as well. His theory that the human body requires either sugar or fat for survival was proved to be true by this diet.

This book covers the reasons why the Atkins diet was

designed. It will also explain the different benefits of following this diet. The main aim might be weight loss, but this is not the only benefit of this diet. When compared to other low-calorie diets, the Atkins diet will facilitate faster weight loss.

The different recipes that are mentioned in this book will ensure that you will be able to consume healthy and tasty food that contains hardly any sugar or carbohydrates. If you are serious about your commitment towards this diet then you will need to set some time aside for procuring all the food that you require for following this diet. This book will definitely make your life easier! There's a list of grocery items that has been provided in this book and you can make use of it while gathering the necessary ingredients. Make sure that you are able to buy the groceries once every week. Motivate yourself to stay on track when you feel like quitting this diet. Do not give in to any temptations and you will definitely live a healthier life.

I would like to thank you once again for purchasing this book. I hope the recipes in this book are enjoyable.

Chapter 1: What is the Atkins Diet?

The Atkins diet is a low-carbohydrate diet and the main objective of this diet is to consume those foods that work well with the metabolism of your body to lose weight. This diet has four phases and it is often combined with exercise for best results.

Dr. Atkins strongly believed that human beings tend to overlook certain factors that are important when it comes to eating habits. These factors are the reason for unnecessary weight gain. The main reason for weight gain is the consumption of processed and refined carbohydrates like sugar.

When you start following the Atkins diet, you will notice that your body is burning up all the excess fat that is stored within your body instead of burning glucose for generating energy. This basic switch in your body metabolism is referred to as ketosis. The insulin level in your body is directly proportional to the level of glucose. A low level of glucose means a low level of insulin. This is when ketosis begins. This means that your body will start burning all the excess fat stored in your body for generating energy only when the glucose level is low.

Usually, your body would have a low level of glucose and insulin prior to eating. Once you consume food, the level of glucose rises and this in turn causes the insulin level to rise as well. When you consume carbohydrates, your blood stream would be full of glucose. There are particular 'good' carbohydrates that have a minimal effect on the glucose levels in your blood. These specific carbohydrates help in the transfer of stored fat from the cells to the blood during ketosis.

Dr. Atkins had stated that a low carbohydrate diet would trigger the metabolism and it will enable your body to burn more calories than it would have on any other diet. During this process, your body also gets rid of the extra calories that it was holding onto.

The term 'Net Carbs' was coined by Dr. Atkins and refers to the total carbohydrates consumed minus all the sugar alcohols and fiber. It was found that the alcohols in sugar don't have any effect on your blood sugar levels. Dr. Atkins truly believed that the carbohydrates with a low glycemic load are the best ones. After thorough research he had come to the conclusion that the consumption of saturated fats should be restricted to about 20% of the total calorie intake.

Four Phases of the Atkins Diet

Phase 1: Induction

The first phase is better known as the induction phase. You will need to make sure that there's a reduction in your daily calorie intake. Once your body has gotten acclimatized to this change, you will need to ensure that your carbohydrate intake has been restricted to only 20 grams per day. Your main source of these carbohydrates would be from vegetables and salads that have low starch content.

In this stage, you prepare your body to burn as much fat as possible. The best way to do so is by consuming very little carbohydrates in order to encourage the body to go after all the fat cells in the body so that they get used as energy. Many people experience a great deal of weight loss during this stage of the diet. But don't worry if you experience medium to low weight loss, as your body will pick up pace as and when you go on with the remaining phases of the diet.

Here is a look at the lifestyle changes you need to make apart from following the meals and foods that are prescribed for the first phase of the diet.

- It is best to stick with your regular meal plan of 3 meals a day or split it into 6 small meals. Make sure that the portions remain the same. It is ideal to limit the carbs to 1 ounce per day.

- Try to incorporate 6 to 8 ounces of proteins during each of your meals. Consume bacon and eggs during breakfast and fish or lean meat during lunch and dinner.

- You can incorporate healthy fats in your diet such as oil, butter and clarified butter. It is a good practice to add about a tablespoon of any of these fats in your meal.

- Remember not to go overboard and starve yourself. If you do so, then you will confuse your body and cause it to stock up on fat. It is therefore important for you to eat on time and consume the prescribed limit of nutrients.

- If you eat lunch out due to work commitments, then it is best to carry your own meals, as eating in an office cafeteria or restaurant might not allow you to customize your meal. If you plan to eat out then it is better to pick a restaurant that serves low carb meals.

- It is important to drink at least 4 ounces of liquids during the first phase of the diet. This can be water, fresh fruit juices, herbal teas etc. It is best to avoid sodas, as they are loaded on dead calories and sugar.

- It is best to make use of a carb calculator to calculate how much you need and whether you are meeting the prescribed limit. If you are over shooting it then you must cut down on it as much as possible.

- It is important for you to take up some form of exercise that will help you shed some extra pounds. Cardio with weights makes for a good workout routine. If you don't have the inclination to hit the gym then walking, swimming or cycling work equally well. Zumba is another fun way to shed them calories.

- The first phase lasts for 2 weeks before commencement of phase 2 of the diet.

Here is a food list that you can consume during the first phase of the Atkins diet.

> Fish such as Cod, Halibut, herring, salmon, sardines, sole, trout and tuna.
> Meats such as Chicken, Cornish Hen, Duck, Goose , Pheasant, Quail, Turkey
> Shellfish such as Clams, Crabmeat, Lobster, Mussels, Oysters, S hrimps and squid.
> Red meats such as Bacon, Beef, Ham, Lamb, Pork, Veal and Venison
> Healthy fats such as Butter, Mayonnaise, Olive oil etc
> Vegetable oils such as Canola, Walnut, Soybean, Grape seed, sunflower oil, sesame oil and Safflower.

Phase 2: Ongoing Weight Loss

The second phase of the diet is known as the ongoing weight loss phase. You will need to add in nutrient and fiber rich food. These are additional sources of carbs and you will need to increase the carb intake to 25 grams during the first week of phase 2 and then keep increasing the intake by five grams every week till you find that there isn't any weight loss. When you reach this stage, you will have to slowly cut down your carb intake by 5 grams till you have reached a stage when you start losing weight once again.

This is the stage where you will notice that you are losing weight faster than the previous stage. The foundation that you lay down during the first phase begins to show results during this phase.

People tend to enjoy this phase the most, as the diet allows the consumption of a variety of foods. Foods that are mostly prohibited during the first phase are allowed to be consumed during phase 2 of the diet. Here is looking at some aspects of phase 2 of the Atkins diet.

- The very first step is to increase the intake of carbohydrates in your diet. The first phase calls for the intake of not any more than 20 grams and the second phase calls for an increase of another 5 grams. You can look up the table and see what foods can be incorporated in the diet to increase the carbohydrate content.

- You have to increase the intake of food in general. For example, if you were consuming 1 cup of vegetable and 1 cup of fruits, then you can increase it to 2 cups of vegetables and 1 and ½ cups of fruits. The same extends to meats, fish, and other foods you are allowed to consume.

- You have to stick with the same amount of proteins that you consumed during phase 1. You can increase it by a little if you like but you must try and keep it at a certain recommended level.

- If you were consuming any multi vitamins during phase 1 of the diet then it is best to continue with them during phase 2. The vitamins will help your body make up for any nutrients that your diet is unable to provide you with.

- It is important for you to remember that you are still on the diet and do not have the flexibility to eat whatever you want. You must stick to the parameters of the diet in order to experience the desired weight loss.

- It is important for you to consume the ideal amount of salt. Salt is important for your body; you can consume foods that are rich in natural salts.

- This stage is known as the ongoing weight loss phase since the weight that you will lose during this phase will be lost for good, provided you stick with the diet for long. If you fall back into your old habits then you will end up putting on the lost weight. It is therefore important to treat this as a permanent phase and consume foods that will help you stave off weight in the long run.

- If you think you are experiencing a good deal of weight loss then stick with whatever meal plan that you are following. If you think otherwise then look into your plan and modify it to experience a positive change in your weight loss journey.

- It will be quite important for you to continue with your exercise regime. You must make an effort to shed the extra weight in your body and burn the excess fat.

- There is no set time frame for phase 2 of the Atkins diet and depends on how much weight you have already lost. The best is to move to the next phase when you are around 10 pounds away from your ideal weight.

Phase 3: Pre Maintenance Stage

The phase 3 of the diet is better known as the pre maintenance phase. This phase is where you maintain the weight loss that you achieved during phase 2 of the diet. As you know, maintaining weight loss is tougher than losing weight and so, this can be considered a tough phase.

You can get started with this phase when you are just ten pounds away from the goal you have set. You can shed those last 10 pounds during this phase and it helps in getting your body fine-tuned to focus on your main health objective.

Here are some things to follow when you are in this phase of the diet.

- It is very important for you to slowly lose the last 10 pounds. Your body should adapt to the weight loss and be able to process the changes. If you hurry the process up then your body will remain confused and not be in a position to change for good. It is ideal to lose the 10 pounds over the course of 4 weeks or so as that will give your body sufficient time to adjust to the changes. You can keep a track of it by checking your weight once a week and ensure that you are on the right course.

- It is best for you to push your threshold a little higher in terms of carb intake. You will, by now, be aware of your threshold and be able to take it up a notch. You can further cut it down depending on how much your body can handle. It will progressively get easier as and when you advance with the diet.

- During this stage of the diet, many people tend to fall off the wagon and roll back to their old habits. This is not such a good thing as your body might start putting back the lost weight. It is therefore important to maintain good control over your cravings and stave off the temptation to consume foods rich in sugars and carbs.

- As mentioned earlier, this stage can prove to be a little tough for you, as you will have to lose weight and keep it from coming back on. For this, you will have to exercise control over yourself and maintain the diet.

- It will be just as important for you to continue exercising, as that is the best way to stave off the excess weight. If you feel dizzy or unable to exercise for long then you can consume a carbohydrate rich meal just before your workout. That way, you will be able to remain with enough and more energy to carry out your workout regime and burn away the carbs that were consumed, when you work out.

- You can go through a food list that is meant specifically for this phase. The foods are all low in carbs and high in other nutrients such as proteins and vitamins. You can try and incorporate them in your regular meals as much as you possibly can.

•   You have to be ready to undertake a fair amount of trial and error to hit upon the right calorie intake for you.

•   At the end of the phase you should have ideally lost your excess weight and reached your desired goal.

•   If you have been consuming multivitamins during the previous two phases then you can consult your physician to reduce the dose. You can also turn to natural supplements such as ashwagandha to maintain the ideal weight.

Phase 4: Lifetime Maintenance

The fourth phase of the diet is known as the lifetime maintenance phase. As you can tell, it refers to maintaining the weight loss that you achieved in the previous 3 stages of the diet. The fourth phase of the diet can be quite tough to carry out and will require mental strength.

You will have to start introducing different sources of carbohydrates at this stage. Monitor your weight closely to avoid any weight gain. If you feel that you are gaining weight, then you will have to do two things. You will have to cut down on the carbs that you are consuming and any new carbs that you might have added to your diet.

You have to be ready to make lifestyle changes that will allow you to stick with the diet for life. Here are some tips to bear in mind.

- Your carbohydrate intake should remain within the prescribed limit. If you have been consuming less than .10 ounce per day, then it is important to stick with that. You must make it a point to count your carbs on a daily basis, as it is important to know how much is being added to your body. A good idea is to maintain a food list and come up with a meal plan that will help you remain within the desired carb limit. Food diaries are often helpful.

- You need not limit yourself to the same foods that you were consuming during the previous two phases. You can experiment with the foods and pick out unique flavors that will leave you feeling healthy and fulfilled.

- You can consume processed foods once in a while but must make sure that you consider it as a treat. You can also consider coming up with healthier options that will help break the monotony and add in a little extra flavor to your diet. Although it is best to avoid the consumption of junk foods as much as possible, you can consider having it once in a while. Add in special flavors that you like in order to spice things up a bit. Be creative!

- Remember not to cut yourself off from all the good things in life. You can still attend parties and enjoy your outings provided you remain a little cautious when it comes to food choices. You can always eat before you leave for the event, carry your own food to such events or tell the host about your dietary restrictions.

- You can continue to consume fats such as butter, clarified butter, nut butters etc. All of these will help your body remain well nourished. Many people make the mistake of cutting these out assuming that it will increase body weight but that is only a misconception; fat is quite important for your body to maintain good health. You can add about a tablespoon of butter to each and every meal, especially the meal that you have before your workout.

- As for the food list, you can make use of the same one that you used in phase 3 and 4. You need not change it, unless you wish for a little variety in your diet.

- You have to continue drinking 8 to 10 glasses of water on a daily basis. You can also drink fresh fruit juices, smoothies and herbal teas to supplement the fluid intake. Consuming a concoction of lemon juice, honey and ginger every morning can help in cutting out the fat in your body and enhance metabolism. You can also add in a little mint to the mixture to enhance its flavor.

- It is important for you to avail at least 8 hours of sleep every night to ensure that your body has the time to heal internally.

- It is best to avoid the intake of alcohol as much as possible. Although it will be impossible to completely eliminate it, you have to try and restraint yourself from letting go. You can consider setting a limit and make sure you adhere to it. The same extends to smoking and recreational drugs. They can tamper with your metabolism and cause you to suffer from weight issues. Once you start with the diet, it will be best for you to not indulge in them or cut them down as much as possible.

- You must also try to stave off stress as much as possible. Stress causes the release of a chemical known as cortisol, which can cause your body to go into panic mode and induce eating disorders. It is therefore extremely important to stave off stress as much as possible and consume foods that help with the process. It is best to eat fiber rich fruits and vegetables, lean meats and fish.

- You can take up yoga and meditation to keep your stress at bay. Indulging in therapeutic activities such as gardening also helps in curbing it to a large extent.

- You can profess about your diet and garner support for the same. Doing so will help you remain motivated and not give up on it as easily. You can also get a partner to join in and together reap the benefits of the diet and motivate each other in the process.

These form the four stages of the Atkins diet. It is best to start as soon as possible and derive lasting benefits.

Chapter 2: Benefits of the Atkins Diet

Weight loss isn't the only benefit of the Atkins diet. The various benefits of following the Atkins diet have been discussed in this chapter.

Epilepsy and Related Diseases

Close to 35 studies that were conducted between 2004 and 2014, have shown that the Atkins diet can help in reducing epilepsy and other seizure disorders in children as well as adults. These studies proved to be encouraging for children who were diagnosed with epilepsy and those who haven't been responding to the medication that was given.

GERD

Studies show that a low-carb diet can help in easing acid reflux. Foods that are fatty or have a high level of caffeine encourage acid reflux. Atkins diet being a low carb diet has a positive effect on GERD.

Acne

A review that was published in Skin Pharmacology and Physiology, after a lot of research, shows that a low carb diet can help in reducing the breaking out of acne.

Heart Diseases

Between the years 2002 and 2014, twenty-one studies were conducted to identify the effect of a low-carb diet on the heart. It was found that such a diet, like the Atkins diet, would help in reducing the risk factor of suffering from heart diseases. It also helps in reducing hypertension and also the levels of cholesterol and triglycerides as well. This helps in preventing inflammation of glands and thereby in controlling the different triggers of heart diseases.

Cancer

Obesity is a factor that is a risk factor for certain types of cancer. It can be inferred that certain types of cancers can be prevented by following a low-carb diet that will help in not only losing but maintaining their ideal weight.

Polycystic Ovary Syndrome

This is a very common problem that affects women in the reproductive age group. This is a problem that's related to obesity, resistance to insulin and hyperinsulinemia. A low-carbohydrate based diet can help in reducing the body's insulin resistance.

Dementia

A high calorific diet is associated with an increase in the risk of damage to the cognitive portion of the brain. A research paper published in 2012 shows that people who consume a high carb diet are at a greater risk of suffering from dementia. The Atkins diet would make sure that this risk could be reduced.

Chapter 3: How to Change Your Mindset to Lose Weight

Reversing the Leadership Model

People who want to lose weight fall into two categories typically. The first category consists of those who would like to fight the battle privately and seclude themselves. The second category consists of the would-be dieter consulting and listening to the nutritionist, doctor, trainer, the author or even the infomercial seller before following a diet. There's nothing wrong with either of the models and they could both work.

The problem comes up only when the follower gets tired of following instructions. Once you get tired of following the strict rules, you would give into your temptations. The problem lies with the dieters. What is required is a well-balanced program of leading and following. You will have to take back some of the control that you have unknowingly passed on to the experts. You needn't do something because that's what your nutritionist asked you to do. You need to realize that you are following the diet for your own good and not for the sake of someone else. You will need to believe in your own cause.

Let Go of Fear

In the world of weight-loss, fear is almost as bad as chocolate pudding. You might fear the weighing scale, the doctor's appointment, shopping for clothes, of taking pictures or of just being simply embarrassed. You are bound to retreat if you start fearing everything. This fear, it's very real and difficult to fight off. Instead of letting this fear control you, you should be able to control your fear.

This is where the concept of setting goals comes into picture. You needn't set big goals; it can be a small goal. Set goals that are attainable. It could be something as simple as abstaining from eating chocolates for a week! You should set a physical and a mental challenge for yourself, something that would scare you to make a good choice, because choices are the means for attaining that goal. Set a challenge and a deadline for overcoming that challenge. This will motivate you to keep going.

Crank Up the Voltage

You need to have a positive mindset if you really want to lose all those excess kilos. Slow and steady wins the race. The choices that you make over a period of time will dictate your progress. Change takes time and it isn't overnight. The same holds true for dieting as well. It is not just about changing your diet; you will have to throw in some exercise into the mix if you really want to reach your weight goal. You will be successful at holding onto a diet only if the diet doesn't feel like a punishment to you. You should enjoy the experience the way a child would enjoy recess. Indulge in physical activities that excite you. The byproduct of truly investing yourself in something is that you will be able to find what you were looking for without any extra effort. If you are really serious about following the Atkins diet, then you will have to change your mind-set a little. Keep trying new recipes, diet doesn't mean bland food. Keep things interesting, on days when you crave for something that you shouldn't eat you can come up with cheat snacks to fulfill your cravings. Don't think of the diet as a punishment, think of it as a means to a healthier life.

Chapter 4: Mistakes to Avoid

The common mistakes that people tend to make while following a diet are discussed in this chapter.

Don't Count Your Total Carbs

You needn't count the total carbs that you consume in a day while following the Atkins diet. You need to count Net Carbs (Total carbs minus the grams of fiber consumed). You shouldn't forget to include the acceptable condiments like lemon juice and various sugar substitutes while calculating your net carbs. Use your carb allowance wisely and don't use it for consuming foods that are rich in sugar and carbs and low in fiber. Don't skip carbs altogether. Make sure that you are consuming the minimum requirement of carbohydrates for your body to function normally.

Skipping Veggies

You shouldn't skimp on vegetables. Make sure that 75% of your minimum carbohydrate consumption is from vegetables. This means that you should eat at least two cups of cooked vegetables and up to 6 cups of leafy vegetables every day.

Saying No to Water

You need to drink at least 8 cups of water daily and this can increase with the increase in physical activity. As long as your urine is pale or clear, it indicates that you are drinking sufficient water. Two cups can be in the form of coffee or tea, broth or sugar-free drinks. It would be a misguided attempt if you skimp on fluids just to see a lower score on the weighing machine. If you don't drink sufficient water, your body will start retaining water as a precautionary measure.

Avoiding Salt

You need to consume a little salt; you shouldn't avoid it. You can avoid headaches, weakness and even muscle cramps by consuming a little salt when your body is transitioning from burning carbohydrates to fat for generating energy. Atkins is a diuretic diet and therefore you needn't avoid salt. However, you should limit your salt intake if you are suffering from hypertension or if you have been advised to do so by your doctor.

Not Eating Sufficient Protein

You will need to consume somewhere between 4 to 6 ounces of protein for each meal, depending upon your age, height and gender. Four ounces might be sufficient for a petite woman but a man might need up to 6 ounces. This doesn't mean that you should consume only protein and skip vegetables, eat too much of protein or vice versa. Doing this will interfere with your weight loss and you will also be subjected to severe cravings for carbs.

Being Scared of Fat

There are certain dietary fats that are essential for the body to burn the fat and these natural fats are fine when you are mindful of your carb intake. You should always accompany a snack of carbohydrates with either fat or protein.

Consuming Hidden Carbs

Read the labels on packaged food items carefully. Just because the package says low calorie, don't assume that it means low carb as well. Make sure that you are using full fat versions of mayonnaise, salad dressings and related products. The low-fat versions tend to mix in additional sugar to replace the flavor that's added by oil.

Becoming a Slave to the Weighing Scale

You should measure and weigh yourself once every week. Your weight tends to naturally vary up to four pounds from one day to another. You will just be setting yourself up for failure if you constantly weigh yourself. This will just cause disappointment and frustration. It is also possible that you are building muscle and shedding fat while working out. This might also cause a slight weight gain and it's perfectly all right. So, your weighing scale might say that you have put on weight whereas you might just be putting on muscle even while your clothes start becoming baggy.

Neglecting to Record Your Progress

You shouldn't neglect to record your progress. Maintain a journal where you are entering all your weekly entries regarding your weight and measurements. You can also include a food journal to keep a track of the carbs you are consuming. Tracking your progress will help you make the necessary changes to your diet so that it would suit your metabolism well.

Chapter 5: Grocery List

Foods to Avoid

- Processed foods that contain sugar, like soft drinks, cakes, chocolates, ice cream and so on.
- Grains like wheat, rye, rice, and barley.
- Vegetable oils like corn oil, canola oil, soybean oil and a few others as well.
- Food items that contain trans-fat or hydrogenated oils.
- So-called "diet" and "low-fat" food products.
- Skip high carb vegetables like potatoes, carrots, turnips, etc. during the induction phase.
- During induction avoid high carb fruits like banana, grapes, oranges and pears
- You should also avoid all legumes during the induction phase.

Foods that You Should Eat

- Make sure that your diet is based on the following food items

- Meats like lamb, chicken, beef, pork, bacon, and turkey.
- Fatty fish like salmon, trout, sardines and other seafood as well.
- Consume eggs because they are rich in Omega 3
- All low-carb vegetables like kale, spinach, broccoli, bell peppers and so on.
- Full-fat dairy products like milk, butter, cream, cheese, and yogurt.
- Nuts and seeds like almonds, cashews, walnuts, sunflower seeds, pumpkin seeds and so on.
- Include healthy fats like olive oil, coconut oil, avocados, etc.

As long as you ensure that your meals are based around any fatty protein and lots of vegetable, some healthy fats and minimal carbohydrates, you will lose weight. It's as simple as that.

Grocery List

Whenever you go shopping for groceries at your local supermarket, it would be advisable that you shop along the perimeter of the store. These are the aisles where they stock up whole foods. You needn't always eat organic produce, but don't opt for processed foods. Select foods that are the least processed and fit into your price range as well.

- Meats like beef, chicken, lamb, pork and bacon.
- Fatty fish like salmon, trout, mackerel and so on.
- Include seafood like prawns and other shellfish.
- Eggs.
- Full fat dairy products like cream, butter cheese, milk, and yogurt.
- Vegetables like spinach, lettuce, kale, broccoli, bell peppers, cauliflower, cabbage, asparagus, onions, Brussels sprouts and so on.
- Fruits like apples, pears, oranges, watermelon, and muskmelon.
- Berries like strawberries, blueberries, raspberries, etc.
- Nuts like cashew nuts, almonds, macadamia, hazelnuts, pistachios, etc.
- Olives.

- Extra virgin olive oil, coconut oil or avocado oil.
- Avocados.
- Dark chocolate comes in handy when you crave for something sweet.
- Various condiments like pepper, sea salt, garlic, chili powder, turmeric, coriander, parsley, etc.

It would really help if you can clear your pantry of all undesirable and unhealthy foods like ice creams, cookies, breakfast cereals, breads, packaged juices and drinks, sugar, etc.

Chapter 6: Atkins Breakfast Recipes

Bacon, Avocado and Jack Cheese Omelet with Salsa (Phase 1)

Ingredients:

- 8 large eggs
- 2 tablespoons butter, unsalted
- 6 slices bacon, cooked, crumbled
- 2 cups Monterey Jack cheese, shredded
- 2 ounces water

For Salsa:

- 1 large ripe tomato, chopped
- 1 jalapeño pepper, finely chopped
- 1 avocado, peeled, pitted, chopped
- 6 medium spring onions, finely chopped
- 2 tablespoons fresh lime juice
- 2 tablespoons fresh cilantro, chopped
- Salt to taste
- Pepper powder to taste

Instructions:

1. To make salsa: Mix together all the ingredients of the salsa and set aside.

2. Whisk together eggs, water, salt and pepper.

3. Place a nonstick skillet over medium heat. Add 1/2-tablespoon butter. When the butter melts, add 1/4 of the egg mixture. Lightly swirl the pan so that the egg spreads.

4. Cook until nearly set. Sprinkle 1/4 each of bacon, avocado and cheese over one half of the omelet. Fold the other half over it. Remove on to a plate and serve.

5. Repeat steps 3 and 4 with the remaining egg mixture and filling.

Scrambled Eggs (Phase 1)

Ingredients:

- 3 large eggs
- 1 tablespoon heavy cream
- Salt to taste
- Pepper powder to taste
- 1 teaspoon fresh parsley, chopped
- 1/2 teaspoon fresh tarragon, chopped
- 1/2 tablespoon unsalted butter

Instructions:

1. Whisk together eggs, cream, salt, pepper, tarragon, and parsley.
2. Place a nonstick skillet over medium heat. Add butter.
3. When the butter melts, add the egg mixture. Cook for a minute. Then scramble it with a wooden spoon. When the eggs are soft and creamy, remove from heat and serve immediately.

Beef Eggs Rancheros (Phase 1)

Ingredients:

- 6 large eggs
- 9 ounces lean ground beef
- 6 slices Canadian bacon
- 3/4 cup canned green chili pepper
- 1 1/2 teaspoons chili powder
- 1/2 teaspoon garlic powder
- 1/2 teaspoon ground cumin
- Salt to taste
- Pepper to taste
- 1/2 teaspoon dried oregano
- 3/4 cup cheddar cheese, shredded
- 2-3 tablespoons fresh cilantro, chopped
- Cooking spray

Instructions:

1. Place a skillet over medium heat. Spray with cooking spray. Add beef and cook until brown.

2. Add chilies, garlic powder, chili powder, cumin, oregano, salt and pepper and cook for another 5-7 minutes.

3. Place the bacon slices on top of the beef and remove from heat.

4. Place a skillet over medium heat. Spray with cooking spray. Add eggs, cook until lightly set and scramble it.

5. To serve: Place a slice of bacon on each plate. Divide the beef mixture into 6 portions and place over the bacon.

6. Divide the scrambled eggs and place over the beef.

7. Sprinkle cheese and cilantro and serve.

Fried Eggs and Vegetables (Phase 1)

Ingredients:
- 4 eggs, beaten
- 1 tablespoon extra virgin olive oil
- 1/2 cup cauliflower florets, chopped into small pieces
- 1/2 cup broccoli florets, chopped into small pieces
- 1 cup spinach, thinly sliced
- Salt to taste
- Pepper to taste
- 1/4 teaspoon chili powder
- 1/2 teaspoon dried oregano

Instructions:
1. Place a nonstick skillet over medium high heat. Add oil. When the oil is heated, add cauliflower and broccoli and sauté for 3-4 minutes.
2. Add eggs, salt, pepper, chili powder and oregano and stir.

3. Add spinach and stir until the eggs are cooked.
4. Serve hot.

Cheesy Tuna Casserole (Phase 1)

Ingredients:

- 3 cans (6 ounce each) tuna, drained
- 24 ounces frozen chopped French green beans, cooked according to instructions on the package
- 5 ounces fresh mushrooms, chopped,
- 2 stalks celery, finely chopped
- 3 tablespoons onion, finely chopped
- 3 tablespoons butter
- 3/4 cup chicken broth
- 1 cup heavy cream or more if required
- Salt to taste
- Pepper powder to taste
- Xanthan gum (optional)
- 8 ounces cheddar cheese, shredded

Instructions:

1. Place a skillet over medium heat. Add butter. When butter melts, add onions and sauté for a couple of minutes. Add

mushrooms and celery and sauté until light brown.

2. Add broth and boil until the broth reduces in quantity by half. Reduce heat and simmer until thick. Stir frequently.

3. Add salt, pepper, tuna, beans and the sautéed mushrooms to a casserole dish.

4. Top with cheese. Bake in a preheated oven at 325° F until the cheese is melted and bubbling.

Baby Spinach Omelet (Phase 1)

Ingredients:

- 4 eggs, whisked well
- 2 cups baby spinach, torn
- 3 tablespoons parmesan, grated
- 1/2 teaspoon onion powder
- 1/4 teaspoon ground nutmeg
- Salt to taste
- Pepper powder to taste
- Cooking spray

Instructions:

1. Add eggs, spinach, and cheese, nutmeg, salt, pepper and onion powder to a bowl and mix well.
2. Place a nonstick pan over medium heat. Spray with cooking spray.
3. Pour the egg mixture and cook until almost set and the underside is golden brown.
4. Flip sides and cook the other side too.
5. Serve hot.

Egg muffins (Phase 2)

Ingredients:

- 10 large eggs, beaten
- 1 medium green bell pepper, diced
- 3/4 cup low fat cheddar cheese
- 3 tablespoons feta cheese
- 1 teaspoon garlic seasoning or to taste

Instructions:

1. Add beaten eggs, green pepper, and garlic seasoning to a bowl and whisk well.
2. Grease muffin molds. Pour the egg mixture (3/4 full) into the muffin molds.
3. Bake in a preheated oven at 325° F for 25-30 minutes or until the muffins are set and browned.
4. Serve hot. They can last for a week if refrigerated.

All Purpose Low Carb Baking Mix (Phase 2)

Ingredients:

- 1/2 cup crude wheat bran
- 10 ounces vanilla whey protein powder
- 10 ounces vital wheat gluten
- 2 1/4 cups whole grain soy flour
- 1/2 cup whole ground golden flaxseed meal

Instructions:

1. Mix together all the ingredients and store in an airtight container. Refrigerate until use. It can store up to a month.

Atkins Cuisine Bread (Phase 2)

Ingredients:

- 2 cups + 1 tablespoon Atkins cuisine all-purpose baking mix - refer recipe 11 further down
- 1 1/2 tablespoons baking powder
- 1/2 teaspoon salt
- 1 packet granular sugar substitute
- 18 tablespoons cold water
- 3 tablespoons vegetable oil

Instructions:

1. Mix together all the dry ingredients in a large bowl.
2. Add water and oil. Use a spatula mix well to form a dough.
3. Take out the dough from the bowl using the spatula and place on a lightly greased, clean work area.
4. Coat your hands with a little oil. Using your hands shape the dough as desired.
5. Place the dough into a greased bread pan.

6. Bake in a preheated oven at 350° F for 1 hour or until done.

7. Remove from oven and place on a wire to cool.

8. Slice only when cooled completely and serve. Store unused bread in an airtight container.

Californian Breakfast Burrito (Phase 2)

Ingredients:

- 6 low carb tortillas, warmed according to the instructions on the package
- 12 large eggs, beaten
- 5 spring onions, thinly sliced
- 1 1/2 tablespoons canola oil
- 6 ounces canned green chili peppers
- 3 tablespoons fresh cilantro, chopped
- 1 large tomato, chopped
- Salt to taste
- Pepper to taste
- 1/4 teaspoon cayenne pepper
- 3/4 cup cheddar cheese, shredded
- Fresh salsa to serve - refer 1st recipe

Instructions:

1. Place a nonstick skillet over medium high heat. Add oil. When the oil is heated, add green onions, tomatoes, salt and pepper and sauté for a couple of minutes.

2. Add eggs and cayenne pepper and stir. Cook until the eggs are done until the consistency you desire. Remove from heat.

3. Place the tortillas on your work area. Divide and place the egg mixture on the tortillas. Sprinkle cilantro and cheese. Add about a tablespoon of fresh salsa.

4. Roll and serve.

Almond Pancakes (Phase 2)

Ingredients

- 1 1/4 cups almond meal
- 4 eggs, separated
- 1 teaspoon baking powder
- Splenda to taste
- 2 tablespoons butter
- 1/2 teaspoon salt

Instructions:

1. Whisk together in a bowl, yolks, cream, and splenda until creamy.
2. Whisk the whites in another bowl until soft peaks are formed.
3. Mix together ground almond and baking and add to the yolk mixture. Whisk well until there are no lumps.
4. Add about 1/4 the whites into the mixture and whisk.
5. Add rest of the whites and fold gently.
6. Place a pan over medium flame. Add about 1/2 tablespoon butter. When butter melts,

add about 1/4 of the batter over the pan at the center. Swirl the pan around so that the batter spreads.

7. Cook until the underside is golden brown. Flip sides and cook the other side too.

8. Repeat the above 2 steps with the remaining batter.

9. Serve warm

Bacon and Egg Casserole (Phase 2)

Ingredients

- 3 bacons
- 4 eggs
- 2 tablespoons green bell pepper
- 1 small onion, chopped
- 4 mushrooms, chopped
- 1/2 cup cheddar cheese
- 4 tablespoons ground flaxseeds
- 1/2 teaspoon salt or to taste
- 1/2 teaspoon pepper powder
- 1/2 teaspoon dried thyme
- 1/3 cup soy milk, unsweetened
- 1 tablespoon olive oil

Instructions:

1. Place a skillet over medium heat.
2. Add oil. When the oil is heated, add onions, pepper, and mushrooms and sauté until onions are translucent.

3. Transfer into a greased baking dish. Spread all over the dish.

4. Layer with cheese followed with bacon.

5. Whisk together eggs, milk, ground flaxseed, thyme, salt and pepper.

6. Pour over the vegetables in the baking dish.

7. Bake in a preheated oven at 350° F until the center begins to set.

8. Switch off the oven and let the dish remain in the oven for 10 minutes before serving.

Almond Soy Mini Muffins (Phase 2)

Ingredients:

- 1 cup unsalted butter, softened
- 1 1/2 cups granulated Splenda
- 1 teaspoon vanilla extract
- 6 eggs
- 1 cup ground almond
- 1 cup soy flour
- 6 teaspoons cinnamon powder
- 1 teaspoon baking powder
- 1/2 teaspoon salt

Instructions:

1. Mix together all the dry ingredients in a large bowl.
2. In another bowl, add butter, vanilla and sweetener. Whip until light and fluffy.
3. Gradually add eggs one by one and beat well.
4. Add the dry ingredients, a little at a time and fold gently.

5. Spoon the batter into lined mini muffin pans (keep it 3/4 full).

6. Bake in a preheated oven at 350° F for about 18-20 minutes or until a toothpick when inserted in the center comes out clean.

Low Carb Porridge (Phase 2)

Ingredients:

- 2 cups coconut or almond milk
- 2 tablespoons sunflower seeds
- 2 tablespoons chia seeds
- 2 tablespoons flaxseeds, whole or crushed
- 1/8 teaspoon salt
- 1/2 teaspoon ground cinnamon
- Fresh berries to serve
- Butter to serve

Instructions:

1. Place a saucepan over medium heat. Add all the ingredients except berries and butter. Stir and bring to the boil.
2. Lower heat and simmer for 2-3 minutes.
3. Remove from heat and serve with butter and berries

Scrambled Tofu (Phase 3)

Ingredients:

- 2 tablespoons olive oil
- 2 bunches green onions, chopped
- 2 cans (14.5 ounce each) peeled, diced tomatoes along with the juice
- 2 packages (12 ounce each) firm silken tofu, drained, mashed
- 1/2 teaspoon ground turmeric
- Salt to taste
- Pepper powder to taste
- 1/2 teaspoon red chili flakes
- 1 cup cheddar cheese, shredded (optional)

Instructions

1. Place a skillet over medium heat. Add oil. When the oil is heated, add green onions. Sauté until tender.
2. Add turmeric, salt and pepper. Sauté for about a minute.

3. Add tofu and tomatoes along with the juice. Mix well.

4. Lower heat and let it heat thoroughly. Sprinkle cheddar cheese if using, and serve.

Acorn Squash with Spiced Applesauce and Maple Drizzle (Phase 3)

Ingredients:

- 2 acorn winter squash (4 inches diameter each), deseeded, chopped into wedges
- 1 1/2 cups apple sauce, unsweetened
- 4 tablespoons butter, unsalted
- 1/4 teaspoon ground cinnamon
- 2 tablespoons sugar free maple syrup
- 1 teaspoon salt
- 1 teaspoon pepper powder

Instructions:

1. Line a baking dish with foil.
2. Melt about 2 tablespoons of butter and brush the squash with it. Season with salt and pepper and place on the baking dish.
3. Bake in a preheated oven at 350° F for about 18-20 minutes or until tender.
4. Meanwhile, add applesauce to a pan and heat it over low flame. Add remaining

butter and cinnamon and cook until well blended.

5. Remove from heat.
6. Serve squash with applesauce. Drizzle a little maple syrup and serve.

Pumpkin Pancakes (Phase 3)

Ingredients:

- 6 large eggs, beaten
- 1/3 cup whole grain soy flour
- 1/3 cup blanched almond flour
- 6 ounces vanilla whey protein
- 1 1/2 teaspoons baking powder
- 1/3 cup curd cream cottage cheese
- 3/4 cup canned pumpkin puree, unsalted
- 3/4 teaspoon pumpkin pie spice
- Butter or canola oil to make pancakes

Instructions:

1. Mix together in a bowl, all the dry ingredients.
2. Add egg, curd cream cottage cheese and pumpkin puree and stir until well combined.
3. Place a nonstick pan over medium heat. Add a little butter. When the butter melts, pour about 1/4 cup of batter on the pan.

Slightly swirl the pan for the batter to spread.

4. Cook until the underside is golden brown. Flip sides and cook the other side too. Remove from the pan and keep warm.

5. Repeat steps 3 and 4 with the remaining batter.

6. Serve warm.

Apple Muffins with Cinnamon - Pecan Streusel (Phase 3)

Ingredients:

- 4 large eggs, beaten
- 3 1/3 cups almond flour
- 4 tablespoons high fiber coconut flour
- 4 tablespoons butter, unsalted, melted
- 1 cup pecans, chopped
- A large pinch stevia
- 16 tablespoons erythritol
- 1/2 cup coconut milk, unsweetened
- 2/3 teaspoon salt
- 4 teaspoons vanilla extract
- 2 teaspoons baking powder
- 1 1/3 cup apple, peeled, cored, finely chopped
- 5 tablespoons ground cinnamon

Instructions:

1. To make pecan streusel: Mix together in a bowl, 1 1/3 cup almond flour, pecans, 4

tablespoons cinnamon, 1/4 teaspoon salt, small pinch stevia, 4 tablespoons erythritol and butter. Mix until a crumbly texture is formed and set aside.

2. To make muffins: Add eggs, coconut milk, vanilla, 12 tablespoons erythritol, small pinch erythritol, and remaining cinnamon to a bowl and whisk well.

3. Add remaining almond flour, coconut flour, remaining salt, and baking powder and mix until well combined.

4. Add apples and fold gently.

5. Pour into lined muffin tins. (Fill up to 1/2). Sprinkle about 2 tablespoons streusel over it.

6. Bake in a preheated oven at 350° F for about 22-25 minutes.

7. Cool for a while and serve.

Bell Pepper Rings filled with Egg and Mozzarella (Phase 4)

Ingredients:

- 4 large eggs
- 1/2 cup mozzarella cheese, shredded
- 1 kiwi fruit, peeled, chopped
- 1/2 cup raspberries
- 1 large banana, sliced
- 1 small apple, cored, chopped
- 1 medium or large bell pepper, sliced into 4 rings of 1 inch each
- 1 tablespoon extra virgin olive oil

Instructions:

1. Place a skillet over medium high heat. Add oil. When the oil is heated, add the bell pepper rings.
2. Break an egg into each of the ring and cook for a couple of minutes.

3. Add about 2 tablespoons water and cook until the egg is set until the softness you desire is achieved.

4. Sprinkle cheese and remove from heat. Cover and set aside for a minute.

5. Meanwhile mix together all the fruits and place on 4 individual serving plates. Place an egg with ring in each plate and serve.

Granola Parfait (Phase 4)

Ingredients:

- 2 cups plain, low fat yogurt
- 2 cups fruits or berries of your choice
- Artificial sweetener or stevia drops to taste
- 1/4 cup rolled oats
- 3/4 cup nuts, chopped
- 2 tablespoons seeds of your choice, toasted
- 1/2 tablespoon olive oil
- 1/2 teaspoon cinnamon
- 1/4 teaspoon vanilla extract
- A pinch of salt

Instructions:

1. In a large bowl mix together the oats, nuts, olive oil, cinnamon, vanilla, salt and a little sweetener.
2. Spread evenly on a greased baking dish.

3. Bake in a preheated oven at 350° F for around 45 minutes, stirring it every 15 minutes.

4. The granola should be golden brown if not then bake further for another 10-15 minutes.

5. To serve: Spoon in the yogurt into glasses. Add some sweetener and stir.

6. Next layer it with fruits and then granola.

7. Repeat the layer. Sprinkle seeds on top. Chill and serve later.

Mexican Potato Omelet (Phase 4)

Ingredients:

- 6 large eggs, well beaten
- 1 1/2 tablespoons olive oil, divided
- 1 red potato (4-5 ounces), rinsed, scrubbed, halved, thinly sliced
- 2 cloves garlic, finely chopped
- 1 cup tomatoes, chopped
- 2 green onions, thinly chopped
- 1/4 teaspoon sea salt or to taste
- 1/4 teaspoon pepper powder or to taste
- 1/3 cup pepper Jack cheese
- 2 tablespoons fresh cilantro, chopped
- 1/2 teaspoon fresh lime juice

Instructions:

1. Add half the oil to a broiler proof skillet and place over medium low heat.
2. Add potatoes, cover and cook until golden brown. Stir occasionally. Add garlic, most

of the scallions, salt and pepper and sauté for about a minute.

3. Add the remaining oil to the pan.

4. Meanwhile, add 1/4-cup tomatoes and 1/4-cup cheese to the eggs and mix well. Pour over the potatoes and cook until the center is almost done.

5. Sprinkle remaining tomatoes, scallions, cilantro, lime juice and cheese over it.

6. Broil in a preheated broiler for 2-3 minutes.

7. Cut into wedges and serve with salsa.

Banana Pancakes (Phase 4)

Ingredients:

- 1 cup almond milk or soy milk
- 4 eggs
- 3 tablespoons butter + extra butter for frying the pancakes
- 2 tablespoons gluten free baking powder
- 2 bananas, pureed
- 1 1/2 cups coconut flour
- 1/2 cup brown rice flour

Instructions:

1. In the food processor bowl, whisk together milk, eggs, and 3 tablespoons butter. Mix well.
2. Add baking powder, coconut flour, rice flour, and bananas until smooth.
3. Heat a non-stick griddle pan over medium heat. Add about a teaspoon of butter. When the butter melts, pour the batter to make small pancakes. Cook until the underside is

golden brown. Flip sides and cook the other side too.

4. Serve warm or hot.

Chapter 7: Lunch / Dinner Recipes

Roasted Red Pepper Soup (Phase 1)

Ingredients:

- 8 ounces roasted bell peppers
- 2 cloves garlic, minced
- 1 small onion, chopped
- 1 stalk celery, chopped
- 1 cup cooked chicken, chopped into bite size pieces
- 4 teaspoons extra virgin olive oil
- 2 cups chicken broth
- 1/3 cup heavy cream
- 1 cup water
- 2 tablespoons parmesan cheese, grated
- Salt to taste
- Pepper powder to taste

Instructions:

1. Place a saucepan over medium heat. Add oil. When the oil is heated, add celery, onions and garlic and sauté until soft.

2. Add roasted peppers, stock and water and bring to the boil.

3. Reduce heat and simmer for 5-6 minutes.

4. Remove from heat and cool for a while. Blend with an immersion blender. Pour the soup back into the saucepan.

5. Reheat the soup. Add cream, salt and pepper and stir. Heat for a couple of minutes more.

6. Serve in soup bowls garnished with cheese.

Cauliflower – Curry Soup (Phase 1)

Ingredients:

- 1/2 tablespoon extra virgin olive oil
- 1 small onion, finely chopped
- 1/2 tablespoon curry powder
- 2 cloves garlic, minced
- 1 inch pieces ginger, grated
- 1 small head cauliflower, cut into small florets
- 1 cup vegetable broth
- 1 cup water
- 1/2 cup heavy cream
- 2 tablespoon fresh chives, chopped
- Salt to taste
- Pepper to taste

Instructions:

1. Place a saucepan over medium heat. Add oil. When the oil is heated, add onions and sauté until translucent. Add curry powder, garlic, and ginger and sauté until fragrant.

2. Add cauliflower, broth, and water. Bring to a boil.

3. Lower heat, cover, and cook until the cauliflower is tender.

4. Add cream. Mix well and remove from heat. Blend the soup with an immersion blender.

5. Pour the soup back to the saucepan and reheat. Add salt and pepper. Heat thoroughly and serve in soup bowls garnished with chives.

Avocado Zucchini Soup (Phase 2)

Ingredients:

- 1 tablespoon extra-virgin olive oil
- 2 green onions, chopped, divided
- 1 teaspoon ginger root, grated
- 1 garlic clove, chopped
- 15 ounce vegetable broth
- 1/2 cup water
- 1 medium zucchini, thinly sliced
- 1/4 teaspoon salt
- Pepper powder to taste
- 1/2 hass avocado, chopped
- 1 tablespoon lemon juice
- 1 tablespoon red bell pepper, chopped

Instructions:

1. Place a large saucepan over medium heat. Add olive oil. Leaving aside 1 tablespoon of the green onion, add the rest to the saucepan. Sauté for 2-3 minutes.

2. Add ginger and garlic. Sauté for a couple of minutes until fragrant. Add vegetable broth, water, zucchini, salt and pepper.

3. Cover and cook for a while until the zucchini is tender. Remove from heat and let it cool for a while.

4. Add avocado. Blend the soup in a blender or with an immersion blender. Transfer the soup back to the saucepan. Reheat the soup and once done, remove from heat.

5. Add lemon juice and red bell pepper. Mix well. Sprinkle the retained green onions.

6. Serve in soup bowls.

Cream of Chicken Soup (Phase 2)

Ingredients:

- 1 cup cooked chicken, chopped
- 4 cloves garlic, minced
- 4 stalks celery, chopped
- 4 cups chicken broth
- 2 tablespoons dehydrated minced onions
- 1 teaspoon dried basil
- 1 teaspoon dried parsley
- Salt to taste
- White pepper powder to taste

Instructions:

1. Add all the ingredients to a food processor and pulse until the consistency you desire is achieved.
2. Place a saucepan over medium high heat. Pour the blended mixture into the saucepan and bring to the boil.
3. Lower heat, cover and simmer for about 20 minutes.
4. Serve in soup bowls.

Soya Bean and Peas Soup (Phase 3)

Ingredients:

- 1/2 cup frozen edamame beans (soya beans)
- 1/2 cup frozen peas
- 1 cup hot vegetable stock
- 3 spring onions, trimmed, chopped
- 1/2 a small bunch basil leaves
- 1 cup light soy milk
- A handful of salad rocket leaves

Instructions:

1. Place a saucepan over medium heat. Add soya beans, peas, stock, and spring onions. Bring to the boil. Simmer for 5 minutes
2. Add basil, rocket leaves, and soymilk. Bring to the boil and remove from heat.
3. Blend half the soup. Pour the blended soup back into the saucepan. Mix well and reheat.
4. Serve hot in soup bowls.

Japanese Vegetables and Tofu Soup (Phase 3)

Ingredients:

- 4 ounces firm tofu, chopped into small cubes
- 4 cups vegetable broth
- 1 1/2 cups bok choy, chopped
- 2 teaspoons ginger, garlic
- 1 Serrano pepper, deseeded, minced
- 1 clove garlic, sliced
- 1 1/2 cups mushrooms, sliced
- 1 medium tomato, chopped
- 1 medium carrot, shredded
- 2 stalks green onion, sliced
- 1 tablespoon fresh cilantro, chopped
- 3 tablespoons Japanese tamari soy sauce
- Salt to taste
- Pepper to taste

Instructions:

1. Place a saucepan over medium heat. Add broth and soy sauce and bring to the boil.
2. Add bok choy, mushrooms, ginger, garlic and Serrano pepper and bring to the boil.
3. Lower heat, cover and simmer for about 5 minutes.
4. Add tomatoes, green onions, tofu and carrot and heat thoroughly.
5. Add cilantro and stir.
6. Serve hot in soup bowls.

Borlotti bean and Kale Soup (Phase 4)

Ingredients:

- 1/2 tablespoon olive oil
- 1 small onion, peeled, diced
- 1 medium carrot, peeled, diced
- 1 medium potato, cut into small chunks
- 1/2 tablespoon tomato puree
- A few sprigs fresh thyme
- 1 bay leaf
- 2 1/2 cups chicken or vegetable stock
- 1 cup canned Borlotti beans, drained, rinsed
- 1 cup curly kale, chopped
- Salt to taste
- Pepper powder to taste
- 2 tablespoons Parmesan, shredded (optional)
- Crusty bread (optional)

Instructions:

1. Place a pan over medium heat. Add oil. When the oil is heated, add onions and carrots and sauté for 3-4 minutes.
2. Add potato, tomato puree, thyme, and bay leaf. Sauté for a couple of minutes and add the stock.
3. Bring to the boil. Reduce heat and simmer for about 10 minutes, cover the pan partially.
4. Add beans, salt, and pepper. Increase the heat back to medium and bring the soup to a boil.
5. Add kale on top; cook until kale wilts.
6. Serve in soup bowls sprinkled with Parmesan with crusty bread if using.

Chicken Pasta Soup (Phase 4)

Ingredients:

- 1 chicken breast (6 ounces), skinless, boneless, chopped into bite sized pieces
- 1/2 cup carrots, cut into matchsticks
- 1 medium onion, chopped
- 2 stalk celery, chopped
- 1 bell pepper, chopped
- 4 cups fat free chicken broth
- Pepper to taste
- Salt to taste
- 1/2 cup whole wheat rotini pasta
- Cooking spray

Instructions:

1. Place a saucepan over medium heat. Spray with cooking spray. Add chicken, onions, celery, carrots, and bell peppers and sauté until the vegetables are tender.
2. Add broth and pasta and bring to the boil.
3. Lower heat and cook until pasta is al dente.
4. Serve hot in soup bowls.

Red Cabbage Slaw with Mustard Vinaigrette (Phase 1)

Ingredients:

- 1 teaspoon lemon zest, grated
- 3/4 pound red cabbage, shredded

For dressing:

- 2 tablespoons extra virgin olive oil
- 1 teaspoon onion, finely minced
- 1/4 cup rice vinegar
- 1 teaspoon prepared mustard
- 1 1/2 tablespoons granulated sweetener

Instructions:

1. Add all the ingredients of the dressing to a salad bowl and whisk until well combined.
2. Add cabbage and toss well.
3. Cover and refrigerate for a couple of hours.
4. Garnish with lemon zest and serve.

Zucchini Pasta Salad (Phase 1)

Ingredients:

- 2 medium yellow zucchinis
- 2 medium green zucchinis
- 2 tablespoons lemon juice
- 1/3 cup parmesan, grated
- Salt to taste
- Pepper powder to taste
- 1 teaspoon lemon zest, grated
- 3 tablespoons olive oil

Instructions:

1. Make noodles of the zucchinis using a spiralizer or julienne peeler.
2. Add all the ingredients to a large bowl and toss well.

Greek Salad with Grilled Chicken Breast (Phase 1)

Ingredients:

- 30 ounces chicken breasts, skinless
- 9 cups romaine lettuce, shredded
- 3/4 cup red onions, sliced
- 18 black olives, pitted
- 2 medium cucumbers, chopped
- 3 medium ripe tomatoes, chopped
- 1 1/2 cups feta cheese, crumbled
- Cooking spray

For dressing:

- 5 tablespoons red wine vinegar
- 1/3 cup extra virgin olive oil
- 1 clove garlic, minced
- 4 teaspoons water
- 3 teaspoons dried oregano
- 1/2 teaspoon salt
- Pepper powder to taste

Instructions:

1. Sprinkle salt and pepper over chicken and set aside for a few minutes.

2. Whisk together all the ingredients of the dressing and set aside.

3. Preheat a grill. Spray chicken with cooking spray and grill the chicken breasts on both the sides until cooked. Remove from the grill, cover and set aside.

4. Add the remaining ingredients of the salad in a bowl. Pour half the dressing and toss well.

5. Divide and place the salad on individual serving plates. Place chicken breasts on top. Pour the remaining dressing over the chicken and serve.

Tuna Salad with Capers (Phase 1)

Ingredients:

- 1 cup Atkins mayonnaise
- 2 cans tuna fish in water, drained
- 2 tablespoons capers
- 4 tablespoons sour cream
- 4 boiled eggs, chopped into bite size pieces
- 4 leeks, finely chopped
- Salt to taste
- Pepper powder to taste
- Chili flakes to taste

Instructions:

1. Add all the ingredients to a bowl and toss well.
2. Serve!

Bacon and Goat Cheese Salad (Phase 2)

Ingredients:

- 4 tablespoons chives, chopped
- 4 cups endives, chopped
- 16 ounces soft goat cheese, cut into slices
- 12 medium slices bacon
- 4 tablespoons extra virgin olive oil
- 3 tablespoons red wine vinegar
- 1-2 large eggs, beaten
- 2 tablespoons Dijon mustard
- 8 cups romaine lettuce, shredded
- 1 teaspoon black pepper powder or to taste
- Salt to taste
- 3 servings Atkins cuisine bread, made into crumbs

Instructions:

1. Place a nonstick skillet over medium heat. Add bacon and cook until crisp. Remove with a slotted spoon and place on paper towels. Crumble when cooled.

2. Retain about 2 tablespoons of the bacon fat and discard the rest.

3. Place bread crumbs on a plate.

4. Dip the goat cheese slices in the egg, one at a time (shake off the excess egg) and dredge in the breadcrumbs.

5. Place the nonstick skillet back on heat. Add a little oil and cook the cheese slices in batches on both the sides until brown. Remove with a slotted spoon and place on paper towels.

6. Meanwhile make the dressing as follows: Add the retained bacon fat, remaining olive oil, vinegar, mustard, and pepper powder to the skillet and whisk well.

7. Place the bacon and greens to a salad bowl. Pour the dressing over the salad and toss well.

8. Divide the salad and place on individual plates. Place a goat cheese patty on each plate and serve.

Asian Beef Salad with Edamame (Phase 2)

Ingredients:

- 2 scallions or spring onions
- 1/2 teaspoon garlic, minced
- 1 tablespoon tamari sauce
- 1/2 teaspoon rice vinegar
- 1/2 teaspoon toasted sesame oil
- 1/4 teaspoon splenda
- 9 ounces beef top sirloin, trimmed of fat
- 1/4 teaspoon curry powder
- 1 teaspoon ginger, ground
- 1 tablespoon canola oil
- 1 1/2 cups spring mix salad
- 1 small red bell pepper, chopped into strips
- 4 ounces water chestnuts
- 1 cup shelled edamame

Instructions:

1. Add to a bowl, green onions, garlic, tamari sauce, rice vinegar, sesame oil, and splenda. Mix well.

2. Pour half of this into a zip lock plastic bag. Keep the remaining half aside.

3. To the zip lock bag, add steak and marinate for 7-8 hours in the refrigerator.

4. Place a large skillet over high heat. Add canola oil. When the oil is very hot, remove beef from the zip lock bag and add to the skillet. Fry until the beef is cooked. Transfer into a large serving bowl.

5. Add mixed greens, bell pepper, water chestnuts, and edamame and mix well.

6. To the other half of the sauce that was kept aside, add curry powder and ginger.

7. Pour this over the salad. Toss well and serve.

Kale Salad (Phase 2)

Ingredients:

- 1 head kale
- 2 cups mixed greens
- 2 cucumbers, peeled and diced
- 4 avocados, peeled, pitted, diced
- 4 tomatoes, diced
- 2 cans garbanzo beans (chickpeas), drained and rinsed
- Topping: hemp seeds or sunflower seeds

For dressing:

- 1 cup tahini
- 1 1/2 cups water + more if required
- 1/4 cup lemon juice
- 2 cloves garlic, minced
- Salt to taste
- Pepper powder, to taste

Instructions:

1. To make the dressing: Add all ingredients of the dressing to a bowl. Whisk well.
2. Add the salad ingredients to a bowl. Pour the dressing over it. Mix well.
3. Chill and serve later.

Avocado Salad with Walnuts (Phase 3)

Ingredients:

- 2 rashers of smoked bacon
- 2 sticks celery, cut into strips lengthwise
- 1 avocado, skinned, diced
- 2 tablespoons walnuts, chopped
- 2 spring onions, cut into strips
- Juice of half a lemon
- 5 tablespoons Atkins mayonnaise
- Mixed leaves salad to serve

Instructions:

1. Preheat a grill. Grill bacon on a wire rack until the bacon is crisp.
2. Mix together celery, avocado, walnuts, spring onions and lemon juice. Add mayonnaise. Toss well.
3. Arrange the salad leaves on a serving platter. Place the salad mixture at the center of the plate.
4. Garnish with bacon and serve.

Chicken Salad (Phase 3)

Ingredients:

- 1 cup chicken, finely shredded
- 1 1/2 tablespoons golden raisins, soak in warm water for about 10 minutes, drained
- 1 tablespoon fresh chives, chopped
- 1 medium carrot, grated
- 4 tablespoons Atkins mayonnaise
- Freshly ground black pepper to taste
- Salt to taste

Instructions:

1. Add all the ingredients to a bowl and mix well.
2. Serve!

Rainbow Salad (Phase 4)

Ingredients:

- 2 large tomatoes
- 3 tablespoons olive oil
- 2 cups baby carrots, chopped into bite size pieces, blanched
- 2 cups cooked whole wheat pasta
- 1 cup basil, chopped, divided
- 1 cup cabbage, shredded
- 1 cup red cabbage, shredded
- 1 cup lettuce, torn
- 2 radish, thinly sliced
- 1 cup fresh mozzarella cheese, cubed

For balsamic dressing:

- 2 ounces olive oil
- 2 ounces white balsamic vinegar
- 2 teaspoons prepared mustard
- Salt to taste
- Pepper to taste

Instructions:

1. Add all the ingredients of the dressing to a jar. Close the lid and shake vigorously and set aside.
2. Add salt, pepper and a little olive oil to mozzarella. Mix well and set aside for a while.
3. Add rest of the ingredients except remaining olive oil and half the basil to a large bowl.
4. Pour dressing and toss well.
5. Place the marinated mozzarella over the salad. Drizzle remaining olive oil over it. Garnish with remaining basil and serve.

Warm Salad (Phase 4)

Ingredients:

- 1/2 cup new potatoes, sliced
- 1 radish, quartered
- 4 cherry tomatoes, halved
- 1/2 tablespoon olive oil
- 1/4 cup haloumi cheese, sliced

For the dressing:

- 2 tablespoons extra virgin olive oil
- 1/2 tablespoon red wine vinegar
- 1/2 tablespoon Dijon mustard
- 2 tablespoons fresh dill, chopped
- Salt to taste
- Pepper to taste

Instructions:

1. Cook the potatoes in boiling water with 1/2-teaspoon salt added to it. When cooked, drain and set aside.

2. Mix together olive oil, vinegar, Dijon mustard, and dill in a large bowl. Add the boiled potatoes, radishes, tomatoes, salt, and pepper. Toss well.

3. Heat a nonstick frying pan with oil. Add haloumi and cook on both the sides until golden brown.

4. Add haloumi to the salad and mix. Divide into individual serving plates.

Mexican Chicken (Phase 1)

Ingredients:

- 1 1/2 chicken breasts, boneless, skinless, cut into strips
- 1/2 green pepper, chopped into 1 inch cubes
- 1/2 red pepper, chopped into 1 inch cubes
- 1 1/2 tablespoon lime juice
- 1 tablespoon chicken broth
- 1/8 teaspoon red chili powder
- 1 teaspoon dried onion
- 1 teaspoon cumin powder
- A large pinch black pepper powder
- 1 clove garlic
- 1/2 tablespoon taco seasoning
- Cheddar cheese for garnishing
- Sour cream for garnishing
- 1 tablespoon butter

Instructions:

1. Mix together limejuice, broth, cumin powder, dried onions, and chili powder in a bowl.
2. Add the chicken strips and toss well.
3. Place a nonstick skillet over medium heat. Add butter.
4. When butter melts, add the chicken pieces, red and green peppers, garlic, pepper powder and taco seasoning. Stir.
5. Cook until the chicken is tender.
6. Transfer on to a microwavable serving platter and top with cheddar cheese. Microwave for about 30 seconds or until the cheese melts.
7. Drizzle sour cream on top and serve.

Bacon and Mushroom Chicken (Phase 1)

Ingredients:

- 4 smoked bacon
- 4 chicken breasts with skin
- 8 tablespoons whipped cream
- 20 mushrooms, quartered
- 2 tablespoons dill, chopped
- 2 cloves garlic, minced
- 1 tablespoon fresh parsley
- 1 1/2 teaspoons salt or to taste
- 1 pound mixed salad greens
- 1 tablespoon butter, melted

Instructions:

1. Grease a baking dish with butter.
2. Sprinkle, salt, garlic, parsley and dill on both sides of the chicken. Place chicken in the baking dish.
3. Place bacon over the chicken followed by a layer of mushrooms

4. Bake in a preheated oven at 350°F for 45 minutes.

5. Pour juices from the baking dish into a bowl. Add cream to it and mix.

6. Pour it over the chicken.

7. Serve chicken with mixed salad greens.

Bahian Halibut (Phase 1)

Ingredients:

- 1 pound Atlantic and Pacific halibut
- 1 tablespoon extra virgin olive oil
- 1/2 cup green sweet pepper, chopped
- 1 small onion, chopped
- 1 small tomato, chopped
- 1 Serrano pepper, deseeded, chopped
- 1 tablespoon lime juice
- 1/2 teaspoon garlic, minced
- 1/4 cup thick coconut milk or coconut cream
- 1/2 teaspoon salt

Instructions:

1. Mix together 1/2-tablespoon oil and limejuice. Dip the fish in it and place on a platter. Set aside.
2. Place a nonstick skillet over medium heat. Add garlic, onion, bell pepper and Serrano

pepper. Sauté until the onions are translucent.

3. Season fish with salt and place the fish in the skillet. Add tomatoes and coconut milk and stir.

4. Lower heat and simmer until the fish is cooked.

5. Taste and adjust the salt if needed. Serve immediately.

Cauliflower "Mashed potatoes" (Phase 1)

Ingredients:

- 2 medium heads of cauliflower or 1 large head cauliflower, cut into florets
- 6 cloves garlic
- 1/4 cup fresh dill, chopped + extra for garnishing
- Sea salt to taste
- Pepper powder to taste
- 1 tablespoon butter
- 2 tablespoons coconut milk

Instructions:

1. Steam the cauliflower, garlic, and broccoli until very soft.
2. Transfer into a bowl
3. Add dill, butter, salt, pepper, and coconut milk. Puree with an immersion blender.
4. Garnish with dill and serve.

Creamy Cheesy Bake (Phase 1)

Ingredients:

- 1 large head cauliflower, chopped into small florets
- 3 cups cheese, shredded
- 16 ounces cream cheese
- 1 cup heavy whipping cream
- 2 pounds frozen or fresh broccoli, boiled, drained
- 4 ounces butter
- Salt to taste
- Pepper powder to taste
- 2 teaspoons garlic powder

Instructions:

1. Add cream cheese, cream, salt, pepper and garlic powder to the boiled broccoli. Blend with an immersion blender until smooth.
2. Grease a baking dish with a little butter. Make small cubes of the remaining butter and place all over the dish.

3. Place the cauliflower florets in the baking dish. Pour the pureed broccoli mixture over the cauliflower.

4. Sprinkle cheese all over the dish.

5. Bake in a preheated oven at 350°F until the cauliflower is tender and the top is golden brown.

Eggplant Gratin (Phase 1)

Ingredients:

- 3 pounds eggplants, cut into 1/2 inch thick slices
- 8 ounces feta cheese
- 3/4 cup cheese, grated
- 3 tablespoons olive oil or butter
- 1/3 cup parsley, finely chopped
- 3 yellow onions, thinly sliced
- 1 1/2 cups heavy whipping cream
- 1 1/2 tablespoons dried mint
- Salt to taste
- Pepper powder to taste

Instructions:

1. Brush olive oil on both the sides of the eggplant slices and place on a lined baking tray.
2. Bake in a preheated oven at 400°F until golden brown.

3. Place a skillet over medium heat. Add oil. When the oil is heated, add onions and sauté until golden brown. Add salt and pepper. Stir and remove from heat.

4. Grease a baking dish with a little oil. Place half the eggplant slices all over the bottom of the dish. Sprinkle half the onions, mint, parsley and about half the feta cheese.

5. Place another layer of eggplant slices and remaining half of the onions. Sprinkle feta cheese and grated cheese. Finally spread whipping cream all over the cheese.

6. Bake at 450°F for about 30 minutes or until the top is brown.

Grilled Steak with Salsa (Phase 2)

Ingredients:

- 1 tablespoon ground cumin
- 2 cloves garlic, minced
- 2 tablespoons lime juice
- 1/2 teaspoon black pepper powder
- 1/4 teaspoon salt
- 3/4 pound flank steak or round
- Fresh salsa to serve - refer 1st recipe in Chapter 6
- Cooking spray

Instructions:

1. Pre heat a grill or broiler rack.
2. Place a skillet over medium heat. Spray the skillet with cooking spray.
3. Add cumin and sauté until fragrant. Transfer into a bowl. Add garlic, 1-tablespoon lime juice, pepper, and salt mix well.

4. Rub this mixture on to the steak well on both the sides.

5. Place in the grill and grill for 5 minutes per side or until cooked.

6. Remove from the grill and cool slightly.

7. Slice the steak into thin slices and serve with salsa.

Asian Tuna Kebabs (Phase 2)

Ingredients:

- 20 ounces tuna, boneless
- 1/2 pound eggplant, chopped into chunks
- 1 medium red bell pepper, chopped into 1 1/2 inches squares
- 2 large scallions, quartered
- 2 teaspoons garlic, minced
- 2 teaspoons ginger, minced
- 2 ounces rice wine
- 1 teaspoon sucralose based sweetener
- 2 teaspoons sesame oil, toasted
- 3 tablespoons tamari or soy sauce
- Salt to taste

Instructions:

1. Soak bamboo skewers in water for 15 minutes before grilling.
2. Preheat a grill to high.
3. Mix together in a bowl, ginger, garlic, soy sauce, rice wine, sesame, ginger, garlic and

sucralose. Add tuna, scallions and red bell pepper. Mix well and set aside to marinate for 15 minutes in the refrigerator.

4. Remove the tuna, scallions and bell pepper from it and thread on to the skewers along with the eggplant in any manner you desire and discard the marinade.

5. Grill for about 3-4 minutes and serve.

Beef Coconut Curry (Phase 2)

Ingredients:

- 1 large onion, chopped
- 1 1/2 pounds grass-fed beef
- 6 cloves garlic, finely chopped
- 1 green bell pepper, chopped
- 1 red bell pepper, chopped
- 2 teaspoons salt or to taste
- Pepper powder to taste
- 2 tablespoons coconut oil
- 3/4 cup tomato paste
- 1 inch fresh ginger, finely grated
- 2 teaspoons ground turmeric
- 2 tablespoons curry powder
- 1 1/2 teaspoons ground cumin
- 1 1/2 teaspoons ground coriander
- 1 teaspoon cayenne pepper or to taste
- 2 cans full fat coconut milk
- 1 head cabbage, sliced
- 2 tablespoons lemon juice

Instructions:

1. Mix together salt, pepper, curry powder, coriander, turmeric, cumin and cayenne pepper in a bowl and set aside.

2. Place a large skillet over medium high heat. Add oil. When oil melts, add onions, bell peppers and garlic and sauté for a couple of minutes.

3. Add beef and cook breaking it simultaneously. Cook until beef is brown.

4. Lower heat. Add tomato paste and ginger and stir. Add spice powder mixture and mix well.

5. Remove from heat. Add coconut milk and limejuice and mix well. Keep warm.

6. To steam cabbage: Place a saucepan filled with water over medium heat. Bring to a boil. Add cabbage and cook until tender.

7. Strain and place on individual serving plates. Serve coconut beef curry over it and serve immediately

Ground Beef and Spinach Skillet (Phase 2)

Ingredients:

- 4 tablespoons coconut oil or ghee
- 2 king oyster mushrooms, chopped
- 4 tablespoons raw almonds, chopped
- 3/4 pound grass fed ground beef
- ½ teaspoon chili pepper flakes
- A large pinch Himalayan salt
- A large pinch ground white pepper
- 1/2 cup pitted kalamata olives
- 2 tablespoons capers
- 2 tablespoons natural roasted almond butter
- 3/4 pound baby spinach leaves, roughly chopped

Instructions:

1. Place a heavy bottomed skillet over medium high heat. Add ghee or oil. When the oil is melted, add mushrooms and sauté until brown.

2. Add almonds and sauté for a minute. Add beef, salt, white pepper powder, chili pepper flakes and cook until the meat is brown and cooked well.

3. Add olives, capers and almond butter. Mix well. Add spinach and sauté for a couple of minutes until the spinach is cooked.

4. Serve immediately.

Cheddar Cheese Open Sandwiches (Phase 2)

Ingredients:

- 2 tablespoons olive oil
- 1 medium red onion, thinly sliced
- 2 tablespoons balsamic vinegar
- 1 teaspoon granular sugar substitute (sucralose)
- 8 ounce sharp cheddar, thinly sliced
- Salt to taste
- Pepper to taste
- 8 slices Atkins cuisine bread, lightly toasted

Instructions:

1. Place a skillet over medium heat. Add oil. When the oil is heated add onions. Sauté until the onions are light brown.
2. Add balsamic vinegar, sugar substitute, salt and pepper. Mix well.
3. Lay the cheese slices over the bread. Divide the onion mixture over the cheese. Spread well.

4. Place in a preheated broiler 4 inches from the heat source and broil until the cheese melts. Serve hot.

Asparagus, Mushrooms & Peas (Phase 3)

Ingredients:

- 1 cup peas
- 2 teaspoons garlic, minced
- 6 ounces Portobello mushroom caps
- 6 medium spring onions, sliced
- 1/2 cup apple cider vinegar
- 2 pounds asparagus
- A handful basil
- Salt to taste
- Pepper to taste
- 6 tablespoons butter, unsalted
- 2 cups water
- 4 tablespoons heavy cream
- 2 tablespoons parmesan cheese, shredded

Instructions:

1. Place a skillet over medium heat. Add 4 tablespoons butter. When the butter melts, add green onions and cook until it wilts.
2. Add garlic and sauté until fragrant.

3. Add remaining butter and mushrooms and cook until mushrooms are tender.

4. Add vinegar and cook for a couple of minutes.

5. Add water and asparagus and bring to the boil. Simmer for 2 minutes.

6. Add peas and simmer until the peas are tender.

7. Add cream and simmer until thick.

8. Remove from heat. Sprinkle Parmesan and serve immediately.

Zucchini Bread (Phase 3)

Ingredients:

- 2 cups almonds, finely ground
- 2 cups soy flour
- 2 cups granular sugar substitute
- 3 teaspoons ground cinnamon
- 1 teaspoon ground nutmeg
- 1 teaspoon salt
- 1 teaspoon baking soda
- 1 teaspoon baking powder
- 1 cup canola oil
- 8 large eggs
- 2 medium zucchini, grated
- 2 teaspoons vanilla extract

Instructions:

1. Mix together all the dry ingredients in a large bowl.
2. In another bowl, add eggs, oil, zucchini, and vanilla extract. Whisk well. Pour this

mixture into the dry mixture bowl. Mix well until the batter is well combined.

3. Transfer the batter into a generously greased bread pan.

4. Bake in a preheated oven at 370° F for about 35 minutes or until a knife comes out clean when inserted

5. Remove from the oven. Cool for 10 minutes and remove from the pan.

6. When cool enough to handle, slice and serve.

Broiled Spicy Orange Chicken Breasts (Phase 3)

Ingredients:

- 3 pounds chicken breast, skinless, quartered
- Salt to taste
- Ground black pepper to taste

For marinating:

- 1/2 cup fresh orange juice
- 4 teaspoons garlic, minced
- 2 tablespoons olive oil
- 2 tablespoons chili powder or to taste
- 2 teaspoons Splenda sweetener
- 2 teaspoons orange rind, grated
- Cayenne pepper to taste

Instructions:

1. Sprinkle salt and pepper over the chicken.
2. Mix together all the ingredients of the marinade. Add chicken and mix well.

3. Transfer the entire contents to a large zip lock plastic bag. Refrigerate for a minimum of 8-7 hours.

4. Preheat a broiler. Place the broiler rack such that it is about 6 inches away from the heating element.

5. Remove from the refrigerator about 30 minutes before broiling.

6. Broil the chicken for about 12-15 minutes or until done. Turn the chicken once while it is cooking.

Spicy Tofu Lettuce Wrap Tacos (Phase 3)

Ingredients:

- 8 ounces extra firm tofu, frozen, thawed, pressed of excess moisture, crumbled
- 2 tablespoons tamari or soy sauce
- 2 teaspoons creamy peanut butter
- 1/2 teaspoon garlic powder
- 1 teaspoon hot sauce
- 1/2 teaspoon ground cumin
- 1/2 teaspoon ground ancho chili
- 1 ripe avocado, peeled, pitted, finely chopped
- 1 head iceberg lettuce
- Fresh salsa to serve - refer 1st recipe in chapter 6

Instructions:

1. Add peanut butter, soy sauce, cumin, garlic powder, chili powder and hot sauce to a microwave safe bowl and microwave for 20 seconds.

2. Remove and mix well. Add tofu and stir.

3. Transfer onto a greased baking sheet.

4. Bake in a preheated oven at 350° F for about 20 minutes.

Chicken Kebabs (Phase 4)

Ingredients:

For the Kebabs:
- 6 chicken fillets, de skinned, cut into chunks
- 1/2 cup low carbohydrate yogurt
- 3 teaspoons ginger paste
- 1/2 teaspoon ground turmeric
- 1/2teaspoon ground coriander
- 1/2 teaspoon ground cumin
- Salt to taste
- Freshly ground pepper to taste

For the Dip:
- 1/3 cup crunchy peanut butter
- 3 tablespoons soy sauce
- 3 tablespoons lime juice
- 1 1/2 teaspoon curry paste
- 1/2 cup low carbohydrate yogurt

Instructions:

1. Mix together all the ingredients of the kebab except chicken and mix well. Add chicken. Coat the chicken with the marinade. Set aside for at least a couple of hours. The longer the better.

2. Thread the chicken kebabs on skewers and grill in a preheated grill for about 10 minutes or until the chicken is cooked.

3. To make the dip: Add all the ingredients of the dip to a blender. Blend until smooth. Transfer into a bowl.

4. Garnish the kebabs with shredded cabbage, onion rings and lemon wedges. Serve the kebabs with the dip.

Garlic Potatoes (Phase 4)

Ingredients:

- 12 medium sized red or Yukon gold potatoes, rinsed, chopped into small cubes with skin on
- 1/4 cup olive oil
- 1 cup soy or almond milk
- Salt to taste
- Pepper powder to taste
- 5 cloves garlic, minced
- 1/3 cup nutritional yeast (optional)

Instructions:

1. Place the potatoes in a large saucepan filled with water. Place the saucepan over high heat and bring to a boil. Cook until the potatoes are tender. Drain the water and place the potatoes in a large bowl.
2. Add rest of the ingredients and mash well and serve with Atkins bread.

Chapter 8: Desserts

Chocolate Peppermint Cupcakes (Phase 1)

Ingredients:

- 1/2 cup coconut milk, unsweetened
- 6 large eggs
- 8 ounces cream cheese
- 14 tablespoons butter, unsalted
- 2 teaspoons vanilla extract
- 1/2 cup xylitol
- 12 tablespoons erythritol, powdered
- 8 tablespoons coconut flour
- 1/2 teaspoon baking powder
- 4 tablespoons cocoa powder, unsweetened
- 1/2 teaspoon salt
- 2 servings peppermint sugar free candy, crushed
- 1/4 teaspoon peppermint extract
- A pinch of stevia (optional)
- Food coloring of your choice (optional)

Instructions:

1. Mix together all the dry ingredients in a bowl.

2. Whisk together eggs, coconut milk, erythritol, vanilla, and peppermint extract and 6 tablespoons melted butter.

3. Add the dry ingredients to it and whisk until well combined.

4. Pour into lined muffin tins (Fill up to 3/4). Line with paper cups.

1. Bake in a preheated oven at 375° F for about 15 minutes or until a toothpick when inserted comes out clean.

5. Remove from the oven. Place on wire racks to cool.

6. Meanwhile make the frosting as follows: Add cream cheese to a bowl and beat until smooth with an electric mixer.

7. Add the remaining erythritol and beat for a minute. Add stevia and food coloring if using.

8. Spread the frosting on top of the cupcakes. Sprinkle peppermint candies and serve.

Chilled Lemon Cheesecake (Phase 1)

Ingredients:

- 2 ounces gelatin powder
- 2 cups water
- 2 pounds cream cheese
- 12 sachets sugar substitute or to taste
- Juice of 2 lemons
- Zest of 2 lemons or to taste
- A large pinch of salt
- Thinly sliced lemon for garnishing
- 1 teaspoon lemon zest, shredded

Instructions:

1. Add water to a saucepan. Sprinkle gelatin powder all over the water. Keep it aside for about 10 minutes to dissolve.
2. Meanwhile add cream cheese and sugar substitute to a bowl. Beat until creamy.
3. Place the saucepan with gelatin over low heat. Stir constantly until the gelatin dissolves. Remove from heat.

4. Pour the gelatin mixture into the cream cheese mixture and beat well.
5. Add lemon juice, lemon zest and salt and blend again.
6. Transfer the beaten mixture into a cake tin. Refrigerate overnight.
7. Garnish with lemon slices and shredded lemon zest.

Decadent Chocolate Ice Cream (Phase 2)

Ingredients:

- 8 large egg
- 4 egg yolks
- 1 1/2 cups cocoa, unsweetened
- 1 teaspoon pure almond extract
- 4 teaspoons vanilla extract
- 6 cups heavy cream
- 1 1/2 cups erythritol or sucralose based sweetener
- 1/2 teaspoon salt

Instructions:

1. Place a heavy bottomed pan over medium heat. Add cream and let it heat for a while. Remove from heat.
2. Whisk together with an electric mixer, eggs, yolks, cocoa, sugar substitute and salt until thick and smooth.

3. Add about a cup of the heated cream and gently whisk. Pour this mixture into the pan of cream whisking simultaneously.

4. Place the pan over medium heat and continue whisking until it thickens slightly. Do not heat beyond 170° F.

5. Remove from heat and transfer into a bowl. Add vanilla and almond extract and whisk again.

6. Refrigerate for at least 2-3 hours. Add the chilled mixture into the ice cream maker and use according to the instructions of the manufacturers.

7. If you prefer soft serve, serve immediately else freeze for 3-4 hours and serve.

Steamed Cinnamon Coconut Milk Egg Custard (Phase 2)

Ingredients:

- 4 eggs
- 4 egg yolks
- 2/3 cup granulated sweetener like splenda
- 4 cups unsweetened coconut milk
- ½ teaspoon ground cinnamon
- 1/2 tsp salt

Instructions:

1. Whisk together eggs and egg yolks in a bowl. Add sweetener and mix well.
2. To another bowl add coconut milk, cinnamon and salt. Whisk well.
3. Pour the coconut milk mixture into the egg yolk mixture. Whisk well.
4. Pour into greased ramekins.
5. Place a baking tray with water in it in a preheated oven. Place the ramekins into a baking tray that is filled with water.

6. Bake in a preheated oven at 300° F for about 30 minutes or until the custard is set.

7. Serve either warm or cold.

Flan (Phase 2)

Ingredients:

- 2 cups heavy cream
- 10 eggs
- 2 cups water
- 2 teaspoons almond extract
- 10 packets sugar substitute or to taste
- 1/2 teaspoon ground cinnamon

Instructions:

1. Add all the ingredients except cinnamon to a blender and blend until smooth.
2. Pour into individual ramekins. Sprinkle cinnamon on top. Place a baking tray with water in it in a preheated oven. Place the ramekins into a baking tray that is filled with water.
3. Bake in a preheated oven at 300° F for about 30 minutes or until the flan is set.
4. Serve either warm or cold.

Fruit Salad (Phase 3)

Ingredients:

- 2 mangoes, peeled, seeded, diced
- 4 pints strawberries, sliced in half
- 2 pints blueberries
- 5 kiwis, peeled, sliced
- 2 pints raspberries
- 4 peaches, diced
- 1 ounce of triple sec
- Juice of 2 lemons
- Juice of 2 oranges
- 1/4 cup mint leaves, for garnish

Instructions:

1. Add all the ingredients to a large bowl. Toss well. Refrigerate and serve chilled garnished with mint leaves.

Pineapple Coconut Granita (Phase 3)

Ingredients:

- 1 whole pineapple, peeled, chopped
- 1 cup water
- 1 cup sucralose sweetener (sugar substitute)
- 1 1/2 teaspoons coconut extract

Instructions:

1. Add pineapple into a blender and blend until smooth.
2. Place a saucepan over high heat. Add sugar substitute and water and simmer until sugar substitute dissolves. Remove from heat. Cool slightly.
3. Add to the blender along with the pineapple and blend until smooth.
4. Transfer into a freezer safe container. Add coconut extract and stir well.
5. Place in the freezer. Remove from the freezer every 30 minutes and break the mixture with a fork. Place it each time in

the freezer. Continue doing this until the mixture is in tiny pieces and frozen as well.

6. When done, cover and freeze until use.

Chocolate Squares (Phase 4)

Ingredients:

- 6 tablespoons butter
- 6 ounces 70 % dark chocolate
- 1 teaspoon vanilla
- 2 teaspoons coffee powder
- 4 ounces creamy peanut butter / almond butter / hazelnut butter
- A pinch salt
- 1/2 cup peanuts / almonds / hazelnuts, roasted, chopped

Instructions:

1. Add butter and chocolate to a microwave safe bowl and microwave until chocolate melts.
2. Add rest of the ingredients except peanuts.
3. Transfer on to a greased and lined baking sheet. Sprinkle the nuts of your choice and let it chill.
4. Chop into 1 inch squares and serve.

Frozen Yogurt Popsicles (Phase 4)

Ingredients:
- 1 pound frozen strawberries
- 1 pound frozen mangoes
- 1 cup heavy whipping cream
- 2 cups low fat Greek yogurt
- 2 teaspoons vanilla

Instructions:
1. Remove the strawberries and mango about 15 minutes before preparing.
2. Add all the ingredients to the blender and blend until smooth.
3. Serve immediately if you prefer soft serve else freeze in an ice cream maker according to the instruction of the manufacturer and serve.

Pineapple Mango Layer Cake (Phase 4)

Ingredients:

- 2 cups soy flour
- 2 teaspoons baking powder
- 1/2 teaspoon salt
- 12 large eggs, separated
- 26 tablespoons granular sugar substitute (sucralose), divided
- 4 teaspoons almond extract
- 1/2 cup unsalted butter, melted and cooled
- 1 cup heavy cream
- 1 pineapple, peeled, cored, thinly slice half the pineapple and chop the other half into small pieces
- 1 mango, thinly slice half the mango and chop the other half into small pieces

Instructions:

1. To make the cake: Mix together soy flour, baking powder and salt in a bowl.

2. Whisk the whites using an electric mixer (keep the speed medium) for a couple of minutes.

3. Add 24 tablespoons of the sugar substitute slowly, beating simultaneously until stiff peaks are formed.

4. To another bowl add yolks, almond extract and butter. Whisk well.

5. With the mixer running, gently pour the yolk mixture into the white mixture. Whisk until well combined. Stop the electric mixer now.

6. Gently fold the flour mixture into the egg mixture.

7. Divide the batter amongst 2 greased baking dishes.

8. Bake in a preheated oven at 350 degree F for about 30 minutes or until a toothpick when inserted comes out clean.

9. Remove from the oven and keep aside to cool for a while. Transfer on to a wire rack to cool completely.

10. To arrange the cake: Add cream and 2 tablespoons sugar substitute to a bowl and whisk well with an electric mixer until soft peaks are formed.

11. Place one of the cakes on a plate. Spoon half the whipped cream over it. Spread it all over the cake.

12. Scatter the mango and pineapple pieces all over the cake.

13. Place the other cake over the mango and pineapple layer. Spread the remaining whipped cream all over the top of the cake.

14. Decorate with sliced mangoes and pineapple.

Slice and serve.

Chapter 9: Smoothies

Detox Green Smoothie (Phase 1)

Ingredients:
- 2 short cucumber, chopped
- 1 cup lettuce leaves, torn
- 2 cups spinach, torn
- 1 cup parsley
- 1/2 cup mint
- 6 stalks celery, chopped
- 2 inch piece fresh ginger, peeled chopped
- 2 tablespoons lemon juice
- 1/2 cup water

Instructions:
1. Add all the ingredients into the blender and blend until smooth. Add more water to dilute the smoothie if you desire a smoothie of thinner consistency.
2. Pour into tall glasses and serve with crushed ice.

Coconut-Vanilla Shake (Phase 1)

Ingredients:

- 4 scoops vanilla whey protein
- 2 cans (14 ounces each) coconut cream
- 1 teaspoon vanilla extract

Instructions:

1. Add all the ingredients into the blender and blend until smooth. Add more water to dilute the smoothie if you desire a smoothie of thinner consistency.
2. Pour into tall glasses and serve with crushed ice.

Spinach Smoothie (Phase 1)

Ingredients:

- 2 scoops vanilla whey protein
- 2 cups spinach, torn
- 3 cups vanilla almond milk
- 1 teaspoon vanilla extract

Instructions:

1. Add all the ingredients into the blender and blend until smooth. Add more milk to dilute the smoothie if you desire a smoothie of thinner consistency.
2. Pour into tall glasses and serve with crushed ice.

Chocolate Smoothie (Phase 1)

Ingredients:

- 2 tablespoons cocoa, unsweetened
- 2 scoops chocolate whey protein
- 1 1/2 tablespoons decaffeinated instant coffee powder
- 6 tablespoons half and half
- 1 cup water
- Ice cubes as required
- Sugar free chocolate syrup (optional)

Instructions:

1. Add all the ingredients into the blender and blend until smooth. Add more water to dilute the smoothie if you desire a smoothie of thinner consistency.
2. Pour into tall glasses. Drizzle sugar free chocolate syrup if using and serve.

Dairy free latte (Phase 1)

Ingredients:

- 4 eggs
- 3 cups hot water
- 4 tablespoons coconut oil
- 1/4 teaspoon vanilla extract
- 1/2 teaspoon ground ginger
- 1/4 teaspoon ground cloves
- 1/4 teaspoon ground cinnamon
- 2 tablespoons cocoa / instant coffee powder

Instructions:

1. Add all the ingredients into the blender and blend until smooth.
2. Pour into tall glasses and serve with crushed ice.

Cucumber Cooler (Phase 1)

Ingredients:

- 2 cups cucumber, peeled, deseeded, chopped
- 1/2 cup fresh mint leaves + extra to garnish
- 2/3 cup water
- 1/2 cup cold water
- Ice cubes as required

Instructions:

1. Add all the ingredients to the blender and blend until smooth.
2. Pour into tall glasses and serve garnished with a mint leaf

Blackberry Smoothie (Phase 2)

Ingredients:

- 2 scoops vanilla whey protein
- 1/2 cup frozen blackberries
- 2 cups vanilla almond milk or coconut milk, unsweetened
- 1 teaspoon vanilla extract
- 2 tablespoons ground golden flaxseed meal
- 1/4 teaspoon ground allspice

Instructions:

1. Add all the ingredients into the blender and blend until smooth. Add more milk to dilute the smoothie if you desire a smoothie of thinner consistency.
2. Pour into tall glasses and serve with crushed ice.

Strawberry Shake (Phase 2)

Ingredients:

- 2 glasses of water
- 2 scoops whey protein powder
- 2 teaspoons bee pollen
- 15 -20 frozen strawberries

Instructions:

1. Blend together all the ingredients until smooth. Transfer into tall glasses.
2. Serve with crushed ice.

Chocolate Peanut Butter Smoothie (Phase 3)

Ingredients:

- 2 scoops chocolate whey protein
- 4 tablespoons natural creamy peanut butter
- 2 cups coconut milk
- 1/8 teaspoon stevia
- 1/2 teaspoon ground cinnamon
- 1/8 teaspoon salt

Instructions:

1. Add all the ingredients into the blender and blend until smooth. Add more milk to dilute the smoothie if you desire a smoothie of thinner consistency.
2. Pour into tall glasses and serve with crushed ice.

Fat burning Green Tea Smoothie (Phase 3)

Ingredients:

- 1 cup broccoli florets
- 1/2 cup cauliflower florets
- 1 cup pineapple pieces
- 1 1/2 cups caffeinated green tea or more according to the consistency you desire

Instructions:

1. Add all the ingredients to the blender and blend until smooth.
2. Pour into tall glasses and serve with crushed ice.

Pineapple Almond Milk Smoothie (Phase 3)

Ingredients:

- 40 whole almonds, blanched
- Ice cubes as required
- 5 ounces fresh pineapple, diced, frozen
- 1 cup low fat Greek yogurt
- 1 cup unsweetened almond milk
- 4 sachets sweetener of your choice or to taste

Instructions:

1. To blanch almonds: Place the almonds in a small saucepan filled with water. Bring to a boil. Simmer for a minute. Drain and rinse with cold water. Remove the skin.
2. Blend together all the ingredients until smooth. Retain a couple of almonds for garnishing.
3. Serve in tall glasses garnished with slivered almonds.

Breakfast Chocolate Smoothie (Phase 3)

Ingredients:

- 3 cups vanilla soy milk
- 3/4 avocado, pitted, peeled, chopped
- 1 1/2 medium banana, peeled, chopped
- 4 tablespoons unsweetened cocoa powder
- 3 individual packets Splenda or any natural sweetener to taste
- Ice cubes as required

Ingredients:

1. Add all the ingredients to a blender and blend until smooth.
2. Pour into tall glasses and serve immediately.

Tropical Fruits Smoothie (Phase 3)

Ingredients:
- 3 cups almond milk
- 1 small banana, peeled, chopped
- 1/2 cup ripe mango, peeled, chopped into chunks
- 1/2 cup frozen pineapple chunks
- 1/2 orange, peeled, seeded, chopped into segments
- 1/2 cup ripe papaya chunks
- 2 tablespoons flax seeds
- 2 tablespoons cashew nuts
- Ice cubes

Instructions:
1. Add all the ingredients to a blender and blend until smooth.
2. Pour into tall glasses and serve immediately.

Kiwi Strawberry Smoothie (Phase 3)

Ingredients:

- 1 cup almond milk or skimmed
- 1 cup low fat plain Greek yogurt
- 1 cup strawberries, chopped
- 1 kiwi, peeled, chopped
- 2 teaspoons orange zest
- 1 teaspoon vanilla extract
- Ice cubes

Instructions:

1. Add all the ingredients to a blender and blend until smooth.
2. Pour into tall glasses and serve immediately.

Breakfast Green Smoothie (Phase 4)

Ingredients:
- 1 medium banana, peeled, chopped
- 4 cups baby spinach, packed
- 2 cups soy milk
- 1/2 cup whole oats
- 2 cups frozen mango
- 1 1/2 cups plain nonfat yogurt
- 1 teaspoon vanilla
- Ice cubes as required

Instructions:
1. Add milk, yogurt, and oats to the blender and blend for about 12-15 seconds.
2. Add rest of the ingredients and blend until smooth.
3. Pour into tall glasses and serve immediately.

Peanut butter Smoothie (Phase 4)

Ingredients:

- 2 tablespoons smooth peanut butter
- 8 ounces plain nonfat Greek yogurt
- 4 cups strawberries, fresh or frozen, chopped
- 1 frozen banana, chopped
- Ice as required

Instructions:

1. Add all the ingredients to the blender and blend until smooth. Add yogurt or water to dilute the smoothie if you desire a smoothie of thinner consistency.
2. Pour into tall glasses and serve.

Mango and Banana Overnight Oats Smoothie (Phase 4)

Ingredients:

For the smoothie:
- 1 ripe banana, peeled, sliced
- 1/2 mango, chopped into chunks
- 1 tablespoon ground flaxseed
- 1 cup almond milk

For the oats:
- 1/3 cup oats
- 1/2 tablespoon ground flaxseed
- 1 small ripe banana
- 3/4 cup almond milk
- 2 tablespoons chia seeds
- Sweetener of your choice

Instructions:
1. Add ingredients of the smoothie into your blender. Blend until smooth.

2. Pour into tall glasses.

3. To make the oats layer: Peel and chop the banana. Add it to the blender along with almond milk, sweetener, and ground flaxseed. Blend until smooth.

4. Add oats and chia seeds. Stir well and pour it over the pureed mango and banana.

Chill in the refrigerator overnight and serve.

Chapter 10: How to Stay Motivated

Understand the Foods that You are Consuming

The Atkins diet is all about consuming such foods that are well suited for your body metabolism. In the previous chapter, you have learned about all such foods that you can and cannot consume. Keep the list in mind whenever you are picking up groceries. You should learn about the foods that will help you shed weight and start cutting down on empty carbs by avoiding sugar. Learn to read labels thoroughly and carefully. Understand the ingredients and read the nutritional facts before you purchase a food product.

Customize Your Diet

The diet plan that you select would depend on the weight that you are trying to lose. The two basic variations of the Atkins diet are the Atkins 20 and the Atkins 40. In Atkins 20 you can consume up to 20 grams of Net Crabs and in Atkins 40 you can consume

40 grams of Net Carbs on a daily basis. Apart from this there are various other food products you can consume and you should make sure that you are following the diet plan that you have selected.

Keep Track of What You Eat

It is quintessential that you keep a track of the amount of carbs that you are consuming while on the Atkins diet. Before you get started with keeping a track of all that you are eating, you will first need to understand the concept of Net Carbs. Net Carbs is different from Total Carbs. You can also make use of various online carb counters for keeping a track of the carbs you are consuming on a daily basis. Make sure that you are sticking to the list of foods that you can consume.

Don't Start Obsessing Over Portions

When you are following the Atkins diet, you needn't have to worry about your calorie consumption. Just make sure that you are allowing your common sense to guide you through the diet. Consumption of calories is extremely important for your well-being, but you shouldn't overdo it. If you consume more calories than what your body is capable of burning, then it will definitely slow down the process of weight loss. But if you cut down on your calorie intake drastically, then it will slow down your metabolism and will hinder weight loss as well.

Don't Starve Yourself

When you are on the Atkins diet, make sure that you keep eating at regular intervals. You can consume five or six small meals trough out the day. Stick to the foods that you can consume and avoid the ones you shouldn't. As long as you are eating what you are allowed to eat and the portions are normal sized, then you needn't worry about your calorie intake. If you starve yourself, your blood sugar levels will drop and it would lead to unnecessary consequences that are perfectly avoidable. If you want to be able to control your appetite and ensure that your energy levels are fine, then you really shouldn't starve yourself. The recipes given in this book will make sure that you have plenty of inspiration to cook healthy and delicious food that will help you curb your craving for carbs.

Include Protein in All Your Meals

You will have to include protein in one form or the other in all your meals. Depending upon your age and gender you will need to consume 4 to 6 ounces of protein on a daily basis. When on the Atkins diet, you can choose from a wide range of proteins, depending on what you fancy. You can consume eggs, fatty meat or even lean meat, seafood and shellfish, any other form of poultry as well. If you like red meat, then you can opt for a fancy marbled cut of beef. Ensure that whatever protein you have opted for, you are cooking it in plenty of olive oil and also that the salads that you are consuming have sufficient dressing as well.

Food that is Naturally Fatty is Good

Fatty food tastes so much better than non-fatty food. Fatty food also tends to fill you up quicker than non-fatty food or lean food. Dietary fat is extremely important when on the Atkins diet. It is essential for maintaining your overall health. But dietary fat doesn't mean trans-fat so steer clear of it. Dietary fat is important for your metabolic functions and skipping fats altogether is a very bad and dangerous idea. Consuming olive oil, full-fat dairy products and even fat cuts of meats will provide you the much-needed dietary fats.

Avoid Sugar at Any Cost

All the soft drinks and other junk food tend to contain a lot of added sugar and this need to be avoided at all costs. All food products that are processed contain added sugars; they are high on calories and low on nutrients. You could opt for non-caloric sweeteners for sweetening your drinks like stevia or sucralose. You will need to ensure that your daily Net Crabs doesn't exceed 3 grams for these non-caloric sweeteners. A simple rule that will help you when you are buying groceries is to stay away from anything that comes in a box.

Consume Lots of Vegetables

You shouldn't skip or cut down on vegetables. Vegetables are good for you and they provide the necessary fiber and nutrients that are required for your body. You will have to make sure that at least 75% of your daily carbohydrate intake comes from vegetables. This means that you can have 5 or 6 servings of vegetables throughout the day. Make sure that you are getting sufficient fiber every day. Fiber helps in controlling the levels of blood sugar in the body. Fiber will also make you feel full and help in maintaining your weight.

Enjoy What You Eat

The Atkins diet is about eating healthy and wholesome foods that are good for you. You will need to enjoy what you are eating and it shouldn't feel like a punishment for you. You don't really have to stock up on expensive pre-cooked meals or anything of that sort. You can eat the regular every day ingredients and the only change that you will be making to your diet is to avoid consuming carbs and sugar. That's all that there is to the Atkins diet. You needn't even worry when you are going out for a meal or travelling. You can order what you want and eat what you want as long as it is an item that this diet provides for. The tasty and nutritious recipes in this book will definitely help you enjoy the diet.

Always Keep Yourself Hydrated

You should keep yourself hydrated to make sure that the electrolyte composition in your body isn't disturbed. You need to drink 8 glasses of water at least and depending on the level of activity that you indulge in, you can drink more water. You can consume a healthy broth or non-caffeinated drinks. Green tea is a good option. If you don't drink sufficient water, it will lead to water retentions. When your body is well hydrated you can get rid of the water weight.

Daily Supplements

When you are on a diet, you should take a few vitamin and nutrient supplements. It is not just about skipping carbohydrates but it is about consuming the right food for your body. Your body needs certain nutrients and if your daily diet doesn't provide those nutrients it can lead to complications. You should consult your nutritionist or your doctor before you decide to take any supplements. The usual supplements that are recommended include supplements for iron, calcium, mineral, potassium, and omega-3and magnesium.

Indulge in Some Physical Activity

Your body metabolism will definitely improve if you indulge in some physical activity. Atkins diet is not just a diet but also a lifestyle choice. If you want to keep the weight that you have lost at bay, then physical activity is as important as following the diet. You needn't necessarily have to go to the gym to exercise, you can go for swimming, brisk walking, and yoga, dancing, Zumba, or you can even play an outdoor game like basketball or tennis. You will not only start burning calories rapidly but will also start building muscle.

Always Keep a Track of Your Progress

It is important that you are keeping a track of your progress. Progress doesn't just mean the weight that you have lost but also the manner in which you have improved your health. Once every week, you should weigh yourself and note down your measurements as well. You should maintain a food journal as well for keeping a track of all that you have been consuming through the day. Record your exercising schedule and any other activity that you think would influence your diet.

Get Support of your Friends and Family

Your family and friends would be your support system. Talk to them about the diet and the dietary restrictions that you have. Get them to understand what you should and shouldn't be doing for your own well-being. When the going gets tough and at times you might also feel like quitting, your family and friends would keep you motivated to keep going.

Plan in Advance

If you are really committed towards following this diet, then it is very important that you plan in advance for all your meals. Your kitchen should be stocked up with all the necessary foods that you can consume while on the Atkins diet. If you don't have the necessary ingredients on hand when you are hungry, it is very likely that you will fall back into your old habits. One thing that you can do is cook in batches and freeze it.

Whenever you have some spare time, you can plan and cook for the next few meals.

Conclusion

I would like to thank you once again for purchasing this book. I hope it proved to be an informational read.

This book provides all the information that you need to know about the Atkins diet. As varied as this diet sounds, it is not just a diet but it's a lifestyle change that will help you in improving your health by working alongside your metabolism and not against it. There are various benefits that this diet offers. You will be able to not only lose weight but also maintain your weight. This diet will make your immune system stronger and your body will be able to avoid many diseases and infections that people these days are being exposed to. You might wonder how you will be able to follow this diet when you are living a fast paced life. But you needn't worry because this book will make following the Atkins diet easy.

The grocery list mentioned in the book will help you gather all the necessary supplies within an hour's time, the low sugar and carb recipes will help you cook delicious and nutritious food, and the simple tricks mentioned will help you stick to the diet.

So, get started right now. It really isn't that difficult, a little bit of extra effort will work wonders for you and you will be able to definitely see a positive change in your body. So get going and the all the best!

Thank you!

Made in the USA
Middletown, DE
16 March 2018